AIR FRYER RECIPES 2021

AFFORDABLE AND SUCCULENT MEAT AND VEGETABLE
RECIPES FOR BEGINNERS AND ADVANCED USERS

SECOND EDITION

JOHN WRIGHT

Table of Contents

Introduction

Are you always looking for easier and more modern ways to cook the best meals for you and all your loved ones?

Are you constantly searching for useful kitchen appliances that will make your work in the kitchen more fun?

Well, you don't need to search anymore! We present to you today the best kitchen appliance available these days on the market: the air fryer!

Air fryers are simply the best kitchen tools for so many reasons. Are you interested in discovering more about air fryers? Then, pay attention next!

First of all, you need to know that air fryers are special and revolutionary kitchen appliances that cook your food using the circulation of hot air. These tools use a special technology called rapid air technology. Therefore, all the food you cook in these fryers is succulent on the inside and perfectly cooked on the outside.

The next thing you need to find out about air fryers is that they allow you to cook, bake, steam and roast pretty much everything you can imagine.

Last but not least, you should know that air fryers help you cook your meals in a much healthier way.
So many people all over the world just fell in love with this great and amazing tool and now it's your turn to become one of them.

So...long story short, we recommend you to purchase an air fryer right away and to get your hands on this cooking journal as soon as possible!

We can assure you that all the meals you cook in your air fryer will taste so good and that everyone will admire your cooking skills from now one!

So, let's get started!
Have fun cooking with your great air fryer!

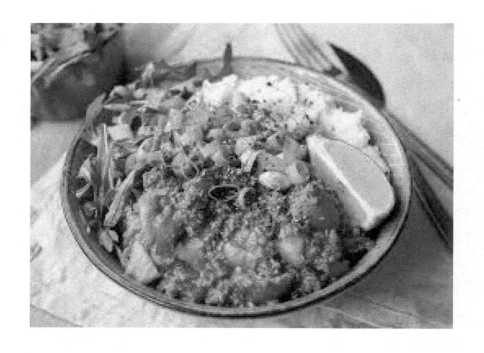

Lamb Roast and Potatoes

Preparation time: 10 minutes **Cooking time:** 45 minutes

Servings: 6

Ingredients:

- 4 pounds lamb roast
- 1 spring rosemary
- 3 garlic cloves, minced
- 6 potatoes, halved
- ½ cup lamb stock
- 4 bay leaves
- Salt and black pepper to the taste

Directions:

1. Put potatoes in a dish that fits your air fryer, add lamb, garlic, rosemary spring, salt, pepper, bay leaves and stock, toss, introduce in your air fryer and cook at 360 degrees F for 45 minutes.
2. Slice lamb, divide among plates and serve with potatoes and cooking juices.

Enjoy!

Nutrition: calories 273, fat 4, fiber 12, carbs 25, protein 29

Lemony Lamb Leg

Preparation time: 10 minutes **Cooking time:** 1 hour **Servings:** 6

Ingredients:

- 4 pounds lamb leg
- 2 tablespoons olive oil
- 2 springs rosemary, chopped
- 2 tablespoons parsley, chopped
- 2 tablespoons oregano, chopped
- Salt and black pepper to the taste
- 1 tablespoon lemon rind, grated
- 3 garlic cloves, minced
- 2 tablespoons lemon juice
- 2 pounds baby potatoes
- 1 cup beef stock

Directions:

1. Make small cuts all over lamb, insert rosemary springs and season with salt and pepper.
2. In a bowl, mix 1 tablespoon oil with oregano, parsley, garlic, lemon juice and rind, stir and rub lamb with this mix.
3. Heat up a pan that fits your air fryer with the rest of the oil over medium high heat, add potatoes, stir and cook for 3 minutes.
4. Add lamb and stock, stir, introduce in your air fryer and cook at 360 degrees F for 1 hour.
5. Divide everything on plates and serve.

Enjoy!

Nutrition: calories 264, fat 4, fiber 12, carbs 27, protein 32

Beef Curry

Preparation time: 10 minutes **Cooking time:** 45 minutes
Servings: 4

Ingredients:
- 2 pounds beef steak, cubed
- 2 tablespoons olive oil
- 3 potatoes, cubed
- 1 tablespoon wine mustard
- 2 and ½ tablespoons curry powder
- 2 yellow onions, chopped
- 2 garlic cloves, minced
- 10 ounces canned coconut milk
- 2 tablespoons tomato sauce
- Salt and black pepper to the taste

Directions:

1. Heat up a pan that fits your air fryer with the oil over medium high heat, add onions and garlic, stir and cook for 4 minutes.
2. Add potatoes and mustard, stir and cook for 1 minute.
3. Add beef, curry powder, salt, pepper, coconut milk and tomato sauce, stir, transfer to your air fryer and cook at 360 degrees F for 40 minutes.
4. Divide into bowls and serve.

Enjoy!

Nutrition: calories 432, fat 16, fiber 4, carbs 20, protein 27

Beef Roast and Wine Sauce

Preparation time: 10 minutes **Cooking time:** 45 minutes

Servings: 6

Ingredients:

- 3 pounds beef roast
- Salt and black pepper to the taste
- 17 ounces beef stock
- 3 ounces red wine
- ½ teaspoon chicken salt
- ½ teaspoon smoked paprika
- 1 yellow onion, chopped
- 4 garlic cloves, minced
- 3 carrots, chopped
- 5 potatoes, chopped

Directions:

1. In a bowl, mix salt, pepper, chicken salt and paprika, stir, rub beef with this mix and put it in a big pan that fits your air fryer.
2. Add onion, garlic, stock, wine, potatoes and carrots, introduce in your air fryer and cook at 360 degrees F for 45 minutes.
3. Divide everything on plates and serve.

Enjoy!

Nutrition: calories 304, fat 20, fiber 7, carbs 20, protein 32

Beef and Cabbage Mix

Preparation time: 10 minutes **Cooking time:** 40 minutes
Servings: 6

Ingredients:

- 2 and ½ pounds beef brisket
- 1 cup beef stock
- 2 bay leaves
- 3 garlic cloves, chopped
- 4 carrots, chopped
- 1 cabbage head, cut into medium wedges
- Salt and black pepper to the taste
- 3 turnips, cut into quarters

Directions:

1. Put beef brisket and stock in a large pan that fits your air fryer, season beef with salt and pepper, add garlic and bay leaves, carrots, cabbage, potatoes and turnips, toss, introduce in your air fryer and cook at 360 degrees F and cook for 40 minutes.
2. Divide among plates and serve.

Enjoy!

Nutrition: calories 353, fat 16, fiber 7, carbs 20, protein 24

Lamb Shanks and Carrots

Preparation time: 10 minutes **Cooking time:** 45 minutes
Servings: 4

Ingredients:

- 4 lamb shanks
- 2 tablespoons olive oil
- 1 yellow onion, finely chopped
- 6 carrots, roughly chopped
- 2 garlic cloves, minced
- 2 tablespoons tomato paste
- 1 teaspoon oregano, dried
- 1 tomato, roughly chopped
- 2 tablespoons water
- 4 ounces red wine
- Salt and black pepper to the taste

Directions:

1. Season lamb with salt and pepper, rub with oil, put in your air fryer and cook at 360 degrees F for 10 minutes.
2. In a pan that fits your air fryer, mix onion with carrots, garlic, tomato paste, tomato, oregano, wine and water and toss.
3. Add lamb, toss, introduce in your air fryer and cook at 370 degrees F for 35 minutes.
4. Divide everything on plates and serve.

Enjoy!

Nutrition: calories 432, fat 17, fiber 8, carbs 17, protein 43

Tasty Lamb Ribs

Preparation time: 15 minutes **Cooking time:** 40 minutes
Servings: 8

Ingredients:

- 8 lamb ribs
- 4 garlic cloves, minced
- 2 carrots, chopped
- 2 cups veggie stock
- 1 tablespoon rosemary, chopped
- 2 tablespoons extra virgin olive oil
- Salt and black pepper to the taste
- 3 tablespoons white flour

Directions:

1. Season lamb ribs with salt and pepper, rub with oil and garlic, put in preheated air fryer and cook at 360 degrees F for 10 minutes.
2. In a heat proof dish that fits your fryer, mix stock with flour and whisk well.
3. Add rosemary, carrots and lamb ribs, place in your air fryer and cook at 350 degrees F for 30 minutes.
4. Divide lamb mix on plates and serve hot.

Enjoy!

Nutrition: calories 302, fat 7, fiber 2, carbs 22, protein 27

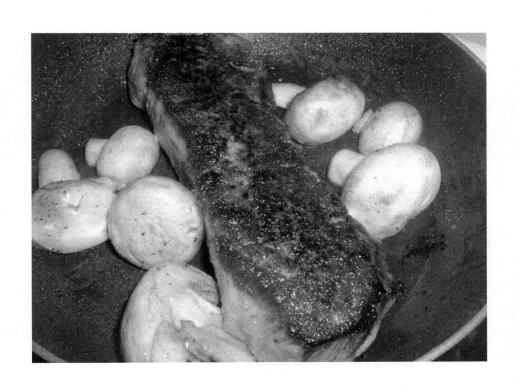

Oriental Air Fried Lamb

Preparation time: 10 minutes **Cooking time:** 42 minutes
Servings: 8

Ingredients:

- 2 and ½ pounds lamb shoulder, chopped
- 3 tablespoons honey
- 3 ounces almonds, peeled and chopped
- 9 ounces plumps, pitted
- 8 ounces veggie stock
- 2 yellow onions, chopped
- 2 garlic cloves, minced
- Salt and black pepper to the tastes
- 1 teaspoon cumin powder
- 1 teaspoon turmeric powder
- 1 teaspoon ginger powder
- 1 teaspoon cinnamon powder
- 3 tablespoons olive oil

Directions:

1. In a bowl, mix cinnamon powder with ginger, cumin, turmeric, garlic, olive oil and lamb, toss to coat, place in your preheated air fryer and cook at 350 degrees F for 8 minutes.
2. Transfer meat to a dish that fits your air fryer, add onions, stock, honey and plums, stir, introduce in your air fryer and cook at 350 degrees F for 35 minutes.
3. Divide everything on plates and serve with almond sprinkled on top.

Enjoy!

Nutrition: calories 432, fat 23, fiber 6, carbs 30, protein 20

Short Ribs and Special Sauce

Preparation time: 10 minutes **Cooking time:** 36 minutes
Servings: 4

Ingredients:

- 2 green onions, chopped
- 1 teaspoon vegetable oil
- 3 garlic cloves, minced
- 3 ginger slices
- 4 pounds short ribs
- ½ cup water
- ½ cup soy sauce
- ¼ cup rice wine
- ¼ cup pear juice
- 2 teaspoons sesame oil

Directions:

1. Heat up a pan that fits your air fryer with the oil over medium heat, add green onions, ginger and garlic, stir and cook for 1 minute.
2. Add ribs, water, wine, soy sauce, sesame oil and pear juice, stir, introduce in your air fryer and cook at 350 degrees F for 35 minutes.
3. Divide ribs and sauce on plates and serve.

Enjoy!

Nutrition: calories 321, fat 12, fiber 4, carbs 20, protein 14

Short Ribs and Beer Sauce

Preparation time: 15 minutes **Cooking time:** 45 minutes
Servings: 6

Ingredients:

- 4 pounds short ribs, cut into small pieces
- 1 yellow onion, chopped
- Salt and black pepper to the taste
- ¼ cup tomato paste
- 1 cup dark beer
- 1 cup chicken stock
- 1 bay leaf
- 6 thyme springs, chopped
- 1 Portobello mushroom, dried

Directions:

1. Heat up a pan that fits your air fryer over medium heat, add tomato paste, onion, stock, beer, mushroom, bay leaves and thyme and bring to a simmer.

2. Add ribs, introduce in your air fryer and cook at 350 degrees F for 40 minutes.

3. Divide everything on plates and serve.

Enjoy!

Nutrition: calories 300, fat 7, fiber 8, carbs 18, protein 23

Roasted Pork Belly and Apple Sauce

Preparation time: 10 minutes **Cooking time:** 40 minutes
Servings: 6

Ingredients:

- 2 tablespoons sugar
- 1 tablespoon lemon juice
- 1 quart water
- 17 ounces apples, cored and cut into wedges
- 2 pounds pork belly, scored
- Salt and black pepper to the taste
- A drizzle of olive oil

Directions:

1. In your blender, mix water with apples, lemon juice and sugar, pulse well, transfer to a bowl, add meat, toss well, drain, put in your air fryer and cook at 400 degrees F for 40 minutes.
2. Pour the sauce in a pot, heat up over medium heat and simmer for 15 minutes.
3. Slice pork belly, divide among plates, drizzle the sauce all over and serve.

Enjoy!

Nutrition: calories 456, fat 34, fiber 4, carbs 10, protein 25

Stuffed Pork Steaks

Preparation time: 10 minutes **Cooking time:** 20 minutes
Servings: 4

Ingredients:

- Zest from 2 limes, grated
- Zest from 1 orange, grated
- Juice from 1 orange
- Juice from 2 limes
- 4 teaspoons garlic, minced
- ¾ cup olive oil
- 1 cup cilantro, chopped
- 1 cup mint, chopped
- 1 teaspoon oregano, dried
- Salt and black pepper to the taste
- 2 teaspoons cumin, ground
- 4 pork loin steaks
- 2 pickles, chopped
- 4 ham slices
- 6 Swiss cheese slices
- 2 tablespoons mustard

Directions:

1. In your food processor, mix lime zest and juice with orange zest and juice, garlic, oil, cilantro, mint, oregano, cumin, salt and pepper and blend well.
2. Season steaks with salt and pepper, place them into a bowl, add marinade and toss to coat.
3. Place steaks on a working surface, divide pickles, cheese, mustard and ham on them, roll and secure with toothpicks.
4. Put stuffed pork steaks in your air fryer and cook at 340 degrees F for 20 minutes.
5. Divide among plates and serve with a side salad.

Enjoy!

Nutrition: calories 270, fat 7, fiber 2, carbs 13, protein 20

Pork Chops and Mushrooms Mix

Preparation time: 10 minutes **Cooking time:** 40 minutes
Servings: 3

Ingredients:

- 8 ounces mushrooms, sliced
- 1 teaspoon garlic powder
- 1 yellow onion, chopped
- 1 cup mayonnaise
- 3 pork chops, boneless
- 1 teaspoon nutmeg
- 1 tablespoon balsamic vinegar
- ½ cup olive oil

Directions:

1. Heat up a pan that fits your air fryer with the oil over medium heat, add mushrooms and onions, stir and cook for 4 minutes.
2. Add pork chops, nutmeg and garlic powder and brown on both sides.
3. Introduce pan your air fryer at 330 degrees F and cook for 30 minutes.
4. Add vinegar and mayo, stir, divide everything on plates and serve.

Enjoy!

Nutrition: calories 600, fat 10, fiber 1, carbs 8, protein 30

Beef Stuffed Squash

Preparation time: 10 minutes **Cooking time:** 40 minutes
Servings: 2

Ingredients:

- 1 spaghetti squash, pricked
- 1 pound beef, ground
- Salt and black pepper to the taste
- 3 garlic cloves, minced
- 1 yellow onion, chopped
- 1 Portobello mushroom, sliced
- 28 ounces canned tomatoes, chopped
- 1 teaspoon oregano, dried
- ¼ teaspoon cayenne pepper
- ½ teaspoon thyme, dried
- 1 green bell pepper, chopped

Directions:

1. Put spaghetti squash in your air fryer, cook at 350 degrees F for 20 minutes, transfer to a cutting board, and cut into halves and discard seeds.

2. Heat up a pan over medium high heat, add meat, garlic, onion and mushroom, stir and cook until meat browns.

3. Add salt, pepper, thyme, oregano, cayenne, tomatoes and green pepper, stir and cook for 10 minutes.

4. Stuff squash with this beef mix, introduce in the fryer and cook at 360 degrees F for 10 minutes.

5. Divide among plates and serve.

Enjoy!

Nutrition: calories 260, fat 7, fiber 2, carbs 14, protein 10

Greek Beef Meatballs Salad

Preparation time: 10 minutes **Cooking time:** 10 minutes
Servings: 6

Ingredients:

- ¼ cup milk
- 17 ounces beef, ground
- 1 yellow onion, grated
- 5 bread slices, cubed
- 1 egg, whisked
- ¼ cup parsley, chopped
- Salt and black pepper to the taste
- 2 garlic cloves, minced
- ¼ cup mint, chopped
- 2 and ½ teaspoons oregano, dried
- 1 tablespoon olive oil
- Cooking spray
- 7 ounces cherry tomatoes, halved
- 1 cup baby spinach
- 1 and ½ tablespoons lemon juice
- 7 ounces Greek yogurt

Directions:

1. Put torn bread in a bowl, add milk, soak for a few minutes, squeeze and transfer to another bowl.
2. Add beef, egg, salt, pepper, oregano, mint, parsley, garlic and onion, stir and shape medium meatballs out of this mix.
3. Spray them with cooking spray, place them in your air fryer and cook at 370 degrees F for 10 minutes.

4. In a salad bowl, mix spinach with cucumber and tomato.
5. Add meatballs, the oil, some salt, pepper, lemon juice and yogurt, toss and serve.

Enjoy!

Nutrition: calories 200, fat 4, fiber 8, carbs 13, protein 27

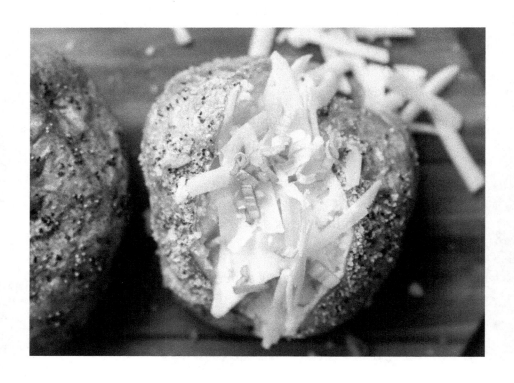

Beef Patties and Mushroom Sauce

Preparation time: 10 minutes **Cooking time:** 25 minutes
Servings: 6

Ingredients:

- 2 pounds beef, ground
- Salt and black pepper to the taste
- ½ teaspoon garlic powder
- 1 tablespoon soy sauce
- ¼ cup beef stock
- ¾ cup flour
- 1 tablespoon parsley, chopped
- 1 tablespoon onion flakes

For the sauce:

- 1 cup yellow onion, chopped
- 2 cups mushrooms, sliced
- 2 tablespoons bacon fat
- 2 tablespoons butter
- ½ teaspoon soy sauce
- ¼ cup sour cream
- ½ cup beef stock
- Salt and black pepper to the taste

41

Directions:

1. In a bowl, mix beef with salt, pepper, garlic powder, 1 tablespoon soy sauce, ¼ cup beef stock, flour, parsley and onion flakes, stir well, shape 6 patties, place them in your air fryer and cook at 350 degrees F for 14 minutes.

2. Meanwhile, heat up a pan with the butter and the bacon fat over medium heat, add mushrooms, stir and cook for 4 minutes.

3. Add onions, stir and cook for 4 minutes more.

4. Add ½ teaspoon soy sauce, sour cream and ½ cup stock, stir well, bring to a simmer and take off heat.

5. Divide beef patties on plates and serve with mushroom sauce on top.

Enjoy!

Nutrition: calories 435, fat 23, fiber 4, carbs 6, protein 32

Beef Casserole

Preparation time: 30 minutes **Cooking time:** 35 minutes
Servings: 12

Ingredients:

- 1 tablespoon olive oil
- 2 pounds beef, ground
- 2 cups eggplant, chopped
- Salt and black pepper to the taste
- 2 teaspoons mustard
- 2 teaspoons gluten free Worcestershire sauce
- 28 ounces canned tomatoes, chopped
- 2 cups mozzarella, grated
- 16 ounces tomato sauce
- 2 tablespoons parsley, chopped
- 1 teaspoon oregano, dried

Directions:

1. In a bowl, mix eggplant with salt, pepper and oil and toss to coat.

2. In another bowl, mix beef with salt, pepper, mustard and Worcestershire sauce, stir well and spread on the bottom of a pan that fits your air fryer.

3. Add eggplant mix, tomatoes, tomato sauce, parsley, oregano and sprinkle mozzarella at the end.

4. Introduce in your air fryer and cook at 360 degrees F for 35 minutes

5. Divide among plates and serve hot.

Enjoy!

Nutrition: calories 200, fat 12, fiber 2, carbs 16, protein 15

Lamb and Spinach Mix

Preparation time: 10 minutes **Cooking time:** 35 minutes
Servings: 6

Ingredients:

- 2 tablespoons ginger, grated
- 2 garlic cloves, minced
- 2 teaspoons cardamom, ground
- 1 red onion, chopped
- 1 pound lamb meat, cubed
- 2 teaspoons cumin powder
- 1 teaspoon garam masala
- ½ teaspoon chili powder
- 1 teaspoon turmeric
- 2 teaspoons coriander, ground
- 1 pound spinach
- 14 ounces canned tomatoes, chopped

Directions:

1. In a heat proof dish that fits your air fryer, mix lamb with spinach, tomatoes, ginger, garlic, onion, cardamom, cloves, cumin, garam masala, chili, turmeric and coriander, stir, introduce in preheated air fryer and cook at 360 degrees F for 35 minutes
2. Divide into bowls and serve.

Enjoy!

Nutrition: calories 160, fat 6, fiber 3, carbs 17, protein 20

Lamb and Lemon Sauce

Preparation time: 10 minutes **Cooking time:** 30 minutes

Servings: 4

Ingredients:

- 2 lamb shanks
- Salt and black pepper to the taste
- 2 garlic cloves, minced
- 4 tablespoons olive oil
- Juice from ½ lemon
- Zest from ½ lemon
- ½ teaspoon oregano, dried

Directions:

1. Season lamb with salt, pepper, rub with garlic, put in your air fryer and cook at 350 degrees F for 30 minutes.
2. Meanwhile, in a bowl, mix lemon juice with lemon zest, some salt and pepper, the olive oil and oregano and whisk very well.
3. Shred lamb, discard bone, divide among plates, drizzle the lemon dressing all over and serve.

Enjoy!

Nutrition: calories 260, fat 7, fiber 3, carbs 15, protein 12

Lamb and Green Pesto

Preparation time: 1 hour **Cooking time:** 45 minutes **Servings:** 4

Ingredients:

- 1 cup parsley
- 1 cup mint
- 1 small yellow onion, roughly chopped
- 1/3 cup pistachios, chopped
- 1 teaspoon lemon zest, grated
- 5 tablespoons olive oil
- Salt and black pepper to the taste
- 2 pounds lamb riblets
- ½ onion, chopped
- 5 garlic cloves, minced
- Juice from 1 orange

Directions:

1. In your food processor, mix parsley with mint, onion, pistachios, lemon zest, salt, pepper and oil and blend very well.
2. Rub lamb with this mix, place in a bowl, cover and leave in the fridge for 1 hour.
3. Transfer lamb to a baking dish that fits your air fryer, also add garlic, drizzle orange juice and cook in your air fryer at 300 degrees F for 45 minutes.
4. Divide lamb on plates and serve.

Enjoy!

Nutrition: calories 200, fat 4, fiber 6, carbs 15, protein 7

Lamb Rack s and Fennel Mix

Preparation time: 10 minutes **Cooking time:** 16 minutes
Servings: 4

Ingredients:

- 12 ounces lamb racks
- 2 fennel bulbs, sliced
- Salt and black pepper to the taste
- 2 tablespoons olive oil
- 4 figs, cut into halves
- 1/8 cup apple cider vinegar
- 1 tablespoon brown sugar

Directions:

1. In a bowl, mix fennel with figs, vinegar, sugar and oil, toss to coat well, transfer to a baking dish that fits your air fryer, introduce in your air fryer and cook at 350 degrees F for 6 minutes.

2. Season lamb with salt and pepper, add to the baking dish with the fennel mix and air fry for 10 minutes more.

3. Divide everything on plates and serve.

Enjoy!

Nutrition: calories 240, fat 9, fiber 3, carbs 15, protein 12

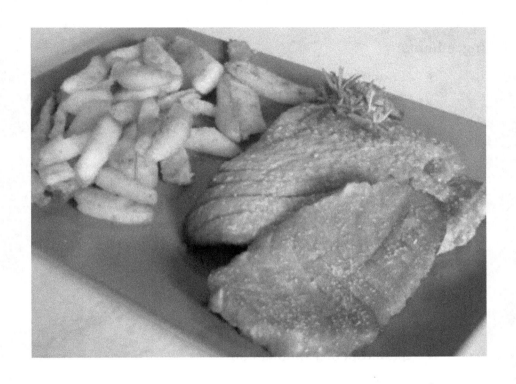

Burgundy Beef Mix

Preparation time: 10 minutes **Cooking time:** 1 hour **Servings:** 7

Ingredients:

- 2 pounds beef chuck roast, cubed
- 15 ounces canned tomatoes, chopped
- 4 carrots, chopped
- Salt and black pepper to the taste
- ½ pounds mushrooms, sliced
- 2 celery ribs, chopped
- 2 yellow onions, chopped
- 1 cup beef stock
- 1 tablespoon thyme, chopped
- ½ teaspoon mustard powder
- 3 tablespoons almond flour
- 1 cup water

Directions:

1. Heat up a heat proof pot that fits your air fryer over medium high heat, add beef, stir and brown them for a couple of minutes.
2. Add tomatoes, mushrooms, onions, carrots, celery, salt, pepper mustard, stock and thyme and stir.
3. In a bowl mix water with flour, stir well, add this to the pot, toss, introduce in your air fryer and cook at 300 degrees F for 1 hour.
4. Divide into bowls and serve.

Enjoy!

Nutrition: calories 275, fat 13, fiber 4, carbs 17, protein 28

Mexican Beef Mix

Preparation time: 10 minutes **Cooking time:** 1 hour and 10 minutes **Servings:** 8

Ingredients:

- 2 yellow onions, chopped
- 2 tablespoons olive oil
- 2 pounds beef roast, cubed
- 2 green bell peppers, chopped
- 1 habanero pepper, chopped
- 4 jalapenos, chopped
- 14 ounces canned tomatoes, chopped
- 2 tablespoons cilantro, chopped
- 6 garlic cloves, minced
- ½ cup water
- Salt and black pepper to the taste
- 1 and ½ teaspoons cumin, ground
- ½ cup black olives, pitted and chopped
- 1 teaspoon oregano, dried

Directions:

1. In a pan that fits your air fryer, combine beef with oil, green bell peppers, onions, jalapenos, habanero pepper, tomatoes, garlic, water, cilantro, oregano, cumin, salt and pepper, stir, put in your air fryer and cook at 300 degrees F for 1 hour and 10 minutes.
2. Add olives, stir, divide into bowls and serve.

Enjoy!

Nutrition: calories 305, fat 14, fiber 4, carbs 18, protein 25

Creamy Ham and Cauliflower Mix

Preparation time: 10 minutes **Cooking time:** 4 hours **Servings:** 6

Ingredients:

- 8 ounces cheddar cheese, grated
- 4 cups ham, cubed
- 14 ounces chicken stock
- ½ teaspoon garlic powder
- ½ teaspoon onion powder
- Salt and black pepper to the taste
- 4 garlic cloves, minced
- ¼ cup heavy cream
- 16 ounces cauliflower florets

Directions:

1. In a pot that fits your air fryer, mix ham with stock, cheese, cauliflower, garlic powder, onion powder, salt, pepper, garlic and heavy cream, stir, put in your air fryer and cook at 300 degrees F for 1 hour.
2. Divide into bowls and serve.

Enjoy!

Nutrition: calories 320, fat 20, fiber 3, carbs 16, protein 23

Air Fried Sausage and Mushrooms

Preparation time: 10 minutes **Cooking time:** 40 minutes
Servings: 6

Ingredients:

- 3 red bell peppers, chopped
- 2 pounds pork sausage, sliced
- Salt and black pepper to the taste
- 2 pounds Portobello mushrooms, sliced
- 2 sweet onions, chopped
- 1 tablespoon brown sugar
- 1 teaspoon olive oil

Directions:

1. In a baking dish that fits your air fryer, mix sausage slices with oil, salt, pepper, bell pepper, mushrooms, onion and sugar, toss, introduce in your air fryer and cook at 300 degrees F for 40 minutes.
2. Divide among plates and serve right away.

Enjoy!

Nutrition: calories 130, fat 12, fiber 1, carbs 13, protein 18

Sausage and Kale

Preparation time: 10 minutes **Cooking time:** 20 minutes
Servings: 4

Ingredients:

- 1 cup yellow onion, chopped
- 1 and ½ pound Italian pork sausage, sliced
- ½ cup red bell pepper, chopped
- Salt and black pepper to the taste
- 5 pounds kale, chopped
- 1 teaspoon garlic, minced
- ¼ cup red hot chili pepper, chopped
- 1 cup water

Directions:

1. In a pan that fits your air fryer, mix sausage with onion, bell pepper, salt, pepper, kale, garlic, water and chili pepper, toss, introduce in preheated air fryer and cook at 300 degrees F for 20 minutes.
2. Divide everything on plates and serve.

Enjoy!

Nutrition: calories 150, fat 4, fiber 1, carbs 12, protein 14

Sirloin Steaks and Pico De Gallo

Preparation time: 10 minutes **Cooking time:** 10 minutes
Servings: 4

Ingredients:

- 2 tablespoons chili powder
- 4 medium sirloin steaks
- 1 teaspoon cumin, ground
- ½ tablespoon sweet paprika
- 1 teaspoon onion powder
- 1 teaspoon garlic powder
- Salt and black pepper to the taste

For the Pico de gallo:

- 1 small red onion, chopped
- 2 tomatoes, chopped
- 2 garlic cloves, minced
- 2 tablespoons lime juice
- 1 small green bell pepper, chopped
- 1 jalapeno, chopped
- ¼ cup cilantro, chopped
- ¼ teaspoon cumin, ground

Directions:

1. In a bowl, mix chili powder with a pinch of salt, black pepper, onion powder, garlic powder, paprika and 1 teaspoon cumin, stir well, season steaks with this mix, put them in your air fryer and cook at 360 degrees F for 10 minutes.
2. In a bowl, mix red onion with tomatoes, garlic, lime juice, bell pepper, jalapeno, cilantro, black pepper to the taste and ¼ teaspoon cumin and toss.
3. Top steaks with this mix and serve right away

Enjoy!

Nutrition: calories 200, fat 12, fiber 4, carbs 15, protein 18

Coffee Flavored Steaks

Preparation time: 10 minutes **Cooking time:** 15 minutes
Servings: 4

Ingredients:

- 1 and ½ tablespoons coffee, ground
- 4 rib eye steaks
- ½ tablespoon sweet paprika
- 2 tablespoons chili powder
- 2 teaspoons garlic powder
- 2 teaspoons onion powder
- ¼ teaspoon ginger, ground
- ¼ teaspoon, coriander, ground
- A pinch of cayenne pepper
- Black pepper to the taste

Directions:

1. In a bowl, mix coffee with paprika, chili powder, garlic powder, onion powder, ginger, coriander, cayenne and black pepper, stir, rub steaks with this mix, put in preheated air fryer and cook at 360 degrees F for 15 minutes.
2. Divide steaks on plates and serve with a side salad.

Enjoy!

Nutrition: calories 160, fat 10, fiber 8, carbs 14, protein 12

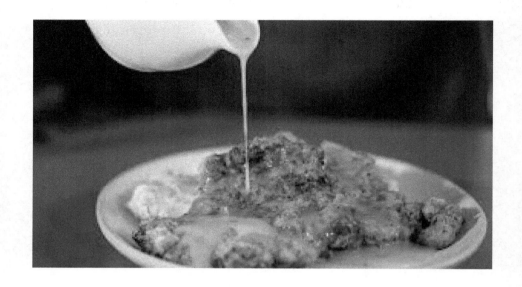

Filet Mignon and Mushrooms Sauce

Preparation time: 10 minutes **Cooking time:** 25 minutes

Servings: 4

Ingredients:

- 12 mushrooms, sliced
- 1 shallot, chopped
- 4 fillet mignons
- 2 garlic cloves, minced
- 2 tablespoons olive oil
- ¼ cup Dijon mustard
- ¼ cup wine
- 1 and ¼ cup coconut cream
- 2 tablespoons parsley, chopped
- Salt and black pepper to the taste

Directions:

1. Heat up a pan with the oil over medium high heat, add garlic and shallots, stir and cook for 3 minutes.
2. Add mushrooms, stir and cook for 4 minutes more.
3. Add wine, stir and cook until it evaporates.
4. Add coconut cream, mustard, parsley, a pinch of salt and black pepper to the taste, stir, cook for 6 minutes more and take off heat.
5. Season fillets with salt and pepper, put them in your air fryer and cook at 360 degrees F for 10 minutes.
6. Divide fillets on plates and serve with the mushroom sauce on top.

Enjoy!

Nutrition: calories 340, fat 12, fiber 1, carbs 14, protein 23

Beef Kabobs

Preparation time: 10 minutes **Cooking time:** 10 minutes
Servings: 4

Ingredients:

- 2 red bell peppers, chopped
- 2 pounds sirloin steak, cut into medium pieces
- 1 red onion, chopped
- 1 zucchini, sliced
- Juice form 1 lime
- 2 tablespoons chili powder
- 2 tablespoon hot sauce
- ½ tablespoons cumin, ground
- ¼ cup olive oil
- ¼ cup salsa
- Salt and black pepper to the taste

Directions:

1. In a bowl, mix salsa with lime juice, oil, hot sauce, chili powder, cumin, salt and black pepper and whisk well.
2. Divide meat bell peppers, zucchini and onion on skewers, brush kabobs with the salsa mix you made earlier, put them in your preheated air fryer and cook them for 10 minutes at 370 degrees F flipping kabobs halfway.
3. Divide among plates and serve with a side salad.

Enjoy!

Nutrition: calories 170, fat 5, fiber 2, carbs 13, protein 16

Mediterranean Steaks and Scallops

Preparation time: 10 minutes **Cooking time:** 14 minutes

Servings: 2

Ingredients:

- 10 sea scallops
- 2 beef steaks
- 4 garlic cloves, minced
- 1 shallot, chopped
- 2 tablespoons lemon juice
- 2 tablespoons parsley, chopped
- 2 tablespoons basil, chopped
- 1 teaspoon lemon zest
- ¼ cup butter
- ¼ cup veggie stock
- Salt and black pepper to the taste

Directions:

1. Season steaks with salt and pepper, put them in your air fryer, cook at 360 degrees F for 10 minutes and transfer to a pan that fits the fryer.
2. Add shallot, garlic, butter, stock, basil, lemon juice, parsley, lemon zest and scallops, toss everything gently and cook at 360 degrees F for 4 minutes more.
3. Divide steaks and scallops on plates and serve.

Enjoy!

Nutrition: calories 150, fat 2, fiber 2, carbs 14, protein 17

Beef Medallions Mix

Preparation time: 2 hours **Cooking time:** 10 minutes **Servings:** 4

Ingredients:

- 2 teaspoons chili powder
- 1 cup tomatoes, crushed
- 4 beef medallions
- 2 teaspoons onion powder
- 2 tablespoons soy sauce
- Salt and black pepper to the taste
- 1 tablespoon hot pepper
- 2 tablespoons lime juice

Directions:

1. In a bowl, mix tomatoes with hot pepper, soy sauce, chili powder, onion powder, a pinch of salt, black pepper and lime juice and whisk well.
2. Arrange beef medallions in a dish, pour sauce over them, toss and leave them aside for 2 hours.
3. Discard tomato marinade, put beef in your preheated air fryer and cook at 360 degrees F for 10 minutes.
4. Divide steaks on plates and serve with a side salad.

Enjoy!

Nutrition: calories 230, fat 4, fiber 1, carbs 13, protein 14

Balsamic Beef

Preparation time: 10 minutes **Cooking time:** 1 hour **Servings:** 6

Ingredients:

- 1 medium beef roast
- 1 tablespoon Worcestershire sauce
- ½ cup balsamic vinegar
- 1 cup beef stock
- 1 tablespoon honey
- 1 tablespoon soy sauce
- 4 garlic cloves, minced

Directions:

1. In a heat proof dish that fits your air fryer, mix roast with roast with Worcestershire sauce, vinegar, stock, honey, soy sauce and garlic, toss well, introduce in your air fryer and cook at 370 degrees F for 1 hour.
2. Slice roast, divide among plates, drizzle the sauce all over and serve.

Enjoy!

Nutrition: calories 311, fat 7, fiber 12, carbs 20, protein 16

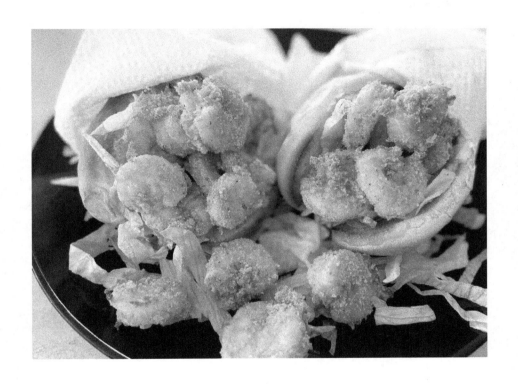

Pork Chops and Roasted Peppers

Preparation time: 10 minutes **Cooking time:** 16 minutes
Servings: 4

Ingredients:

- 3 tablespoons olive oil
- 3 tablespoons lemon juice
- 1 tablespoon smoked paprika
- 2 tablespoons thyme, chopped
- 3 garlic cloves, minced
- 4 pork chops, bone in
- Salta and black pepper to the taste
- 2 roasted bell peppers, chopped

Directions:

1. In a pan that fits your air fryer, mix pork chops with oil, lemon juice, smoked paprika, thyme, garlic, bell peppers, salt and pepper, toss well, introduce in your air fryer and cook at 400 degrees F for 16 minutes.
2. Divide pork chops and peppers mix on plates and serve right away.

Enjoy!

Nutrition: calories 321, fat 6, fiber 8, carbs 14, protein 17

Pork Chops and Green Beans

Preparation time: 10 minutes **Cooking time:** 15 minutes
Servings: 4

Ingredients:

- 4 pork chops, bone in
- 2 tablespoons olive oil
- 1 tablespoon sage, chopped
- Salt and black pepper to the taste
- 16 ounces green beans
- 3 garlic cloves, minced
- 2 tablespoons parsley, chopped

Directions:

1. In a pan that fits your air fryer, mix pork chops with olive oil, sage, salt, pepper, green beans, garlic and parsley, toss, introduce in your air fryer and cook at 360 degrees F for 15 minutes.
2. Divide everything on plates and serve.

Enjoy!

Nutrition: calories 261, fat 7, fiber 9, carbs 14, protein 20

Pork Chops and Sage Sauce

Preparation time: 10 minutes **Cooking time:** 15 minutes

Servings: 2

Ingredients:

- 2 pork chops
- Salt and black pepper to the taste
- 1 tablespoon olive oil
- 2 tablespoons butter
- 1 shallot, sliced
- 1 handful sage, chopped
- 1 teaspoon lemon juice

Directions:

1. Season pork chops with salt and pepper, rub with the oil, put in your air fryer and cook at 370 degrees F for 10 minutes, flipping them halfway.
2. Meanwhile, heat up a pan with the butter over medium heat, add shallot, stir and cook for 2 minutes.
3. Add sage and lemon juice, stir well, cook for a few more minutes and take off heat.
4. Divide pork chops on plates, drizzle sage sauce all over and serve.

Enjoy!

Nutrition: calories 265, fat 6, fiber 8, carbs 19, protein 12

Tasty Ham and Greens

Preparation time: 10 minutes **Cooking time:** 16 minutes
Servings: 8

Ingredients:
- 2 tablespoons olive oil
- 4 cups ham, chopped
- 2 tablespoons flour
- 3 cups chicken stock
- 5 ounces onion, chopped
- 16 ounces collard greens, chopped
- 14 ounces canned black eyed peas, drained
- ½ teaspoon red pepper, crushed

Directions:

1. Drizzle the oil in a pan that fits your air fryer, add ham, stock and flour and whisk.
2. Also add onion, black eyed peas, red pepper and collard greens, introduce in your air fryer and cook at 390 degrees F for 16 minutes.
3. Divide everything on plates and serve.

Enjoy!

Nutrition: calories 322, fat 6, fiber 8, carbs 12, protein 5

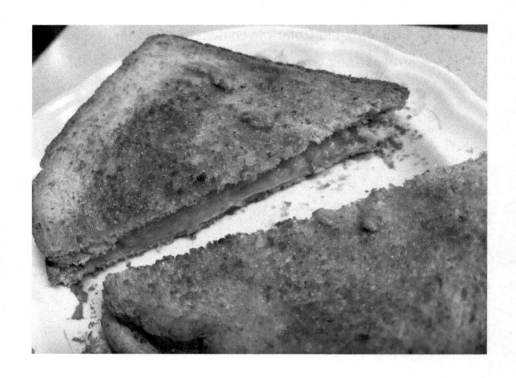

Ham and Veggie Air Fried Mix

Preparation time: 10 minutes **Cooking time:** 20 minutes
Servings: 6

Ingredients:

- ¼ cup butter
- ¼ cup flour
- 3 cups milk
- ½ teaspoon thyme, dried
- 2 cups ham, chopped
- 6 ounces sweet peas
- 4 ounces mushrooms, halved
- 1 cup baby carrots

Directions:

1. Heat up a large pan that fits your air fryer with the butter over medium heat, melt it, add flour and whisk well.
2. Add milk and, well again and take off heat.
3. Add thyme, ham, peas, mushrooms and baby carrots, toss, put in your air fryer and cook at 360 degrees F for 20 minutes.
4. Divide everything on plates and serve.

Enjoy!

Nutrition: calories 311, fat 6, fiber 8, carbs 12, protein 7

Air Fryer Vegetable Recipes

Spinach Pie

Preparation time: 10 minutes **Cooking time:** 15 minutes
Servings: 4

Ingredients:

- 7 ounces flour
- 2 tablespoons butter
- 7 ounces spinach
- 1 tablespoon olive oil
- 2 eggs
- 2 tablespoons milk
- 3 ounces cottage cheese
- Salt and black pepper to the taste
- 1 yellow onion, chopped

Directions:

1. In your food processor, mix flour with butter, 1 egg, milk, salt and pepper, blend well, transfer to a bowl, knead, cover and leave for 10 minutes.
2. Heat up a pan with the oil over medium high heat, add onion and spinach, stir and cook for 2 minutes.
3. Add salt, pepper, the remaining egg and cottage cheese, stir well and take off heat.
4. Divide dough in 4 pieces, roll each piece, place on the bottom of a ramekin, add spinach filling over dough, place ramekins in your air fryer's basket and cook at 360 degrees F for 15 minutes.
5. Serve warm,

Enjoy!

Nutrition: calories 250, fat 12, fiber 2, carbs 23, protein 12

Balsamic Artichokes

Preparation time: 10 minutes **Cooking time:** 7 minutes

Servings: 4

Ingredients:

- 4 big artichokes, trimmed
- Salt and black pepper to the taste
- 2 tablespoons lemon juice
- ¼ cup extra virgin olive oil
- 2 teaspoons balsamic vinegar
- 1 teaspoon oregano, dried
- 2 garlic cloves, minced

Directions:

1. Season artichokes with salt and pepper, rub them with half of the oil and half of the lemon juice, put them in your air fryer and cook at 360 degrees F for 7 minutes.
2. Meanwhile, in a bowl, mix the rest of the lemon juice with vinegar, the remaining oil, salt, pepper, garlic and oregano and stir very well.
3. Arrange artichokes on a platter, drizzle the balsamic vinaigrette over them and serve.

Enjoy!

Nutrition: calories 200, fat 3, fiber 6, carbs 12, protein 4

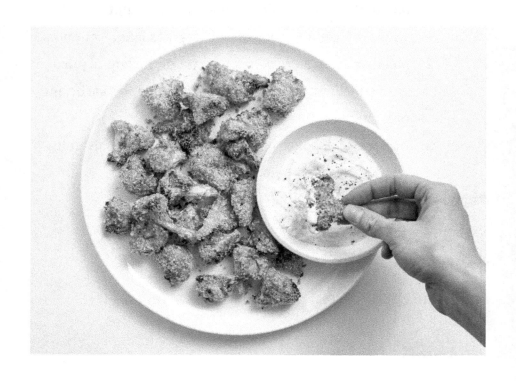

Cheesy Artichokes

Preparation time: 10 minutes **Cooking time:** 6 minutes

Servings: 6

Ingredients:

- 14 ounces canned artichoke hearts
- 8 ounces cream cheese
- 16 ounces parmesan cheese, grated
- 10 ounces spinach
- ½ cup chicken stock
- 8 ounces mozzarella, shredded
- ½ cup sour cream
- 3 garlic cloves, minced
- ½ cup mayonnaise
- 1 teaspoon onion powder

Directions:

1. In a pan that fits your air fryer, mix artichokes with stock, garlic, spinach, cream cheese, sour cream, onion powder and mayo, toss, introduce in your air fryer and cook at 350 degrees F for 6 minutes.
2. Add mozzarella and parmesan, stir well and serve.

Enjoy!

Nutrition: calories 261, fat 12, fiber 2, carbs 12, protein 15

Artichokes and Special Sauce

Preparation time: 10 minutes **Cooking time:** 6 minutes
Servings: 2

Ingredients:

- 2 artichokes, trimmed
- A drizzle of olive oil
- 2 garlic cloves, minced
- 1 tablespoon lemon juice

For the sauce:

- ¼ cup coconut oil
- ¼ cup extra virgin olive oil
- 3 anchovy fillets
- 3 garlic cloves

Directions:

1. In a bowl, mix artichokes with oil, 2 garlic cloves and lemon juice, toss well, transfer to your air fryer, cook at 350 degrees F for 6 minutes and divide among plates.
2. In your food processor, mix coconut oil with anchovy, 3 garlic cloves and olive oil, blend very well, drizzle over artichokes and serve.

Enjoy!

Nutrition: calories 261, fat 4, fiber 7, carbs 20, protein 12

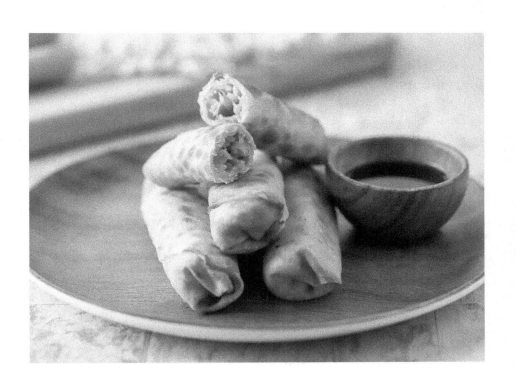

Beet Salad and Parsley Dressing

Preparation time: 10 minutes **Cooking time:** 14 minutes
Servings: 4

Ingredients:

- 4 beets
- 2 tablespoons balsamic vinegar
- A bunch of parsley, chopped
- Salt and black pepper to the taste
- 1 tablespoon extra virgin olive oil
- 1 garlic clove, chopped
- 2 tablespoons capers

Directions:

1. Put beets in your air fryer and cook them at 360 degrees F for 14 minutes.
2. Meanwhile, in a bowl, mix parsley with garlic, salt, pepper, olive oil and capers and stir very well.
3. Transfer beets to a cutting board, leave them to cool down, peel them, slice put them in a salad bowl.
4. Add vinegar, drizzle the parsley dressing all over and serve.

Enjoy!

Nutrition: calories 70, fat 2, fiber 1, carbs 6, protein 4

Beets and Blue Cheese Salad

Preparation time: 10 minutes **Cooking time:** 14 minutes
Servings: 6

Ingredients:

- 6 beets, peeled and quartered
- Salt and black pepper to the taste
- ¼ cup blue cheese, crumbled
- 1 tablespoon olive oil

Directions:

1. Put beets in your air fryer, cook them at 350 degrees F for 14 minutes and transfer them to a bowl.
2. Add blue cheese, salt, pepper and oil, toss and serve.

Enjoy!

Nutrition: calories 100, fat 4, fiber 4, carbs 10, protein 5

Beet s and Arugula Salad

Preparation time: 10 minutes **Cooking time:** 10 minutes

Servings: 4

Ingredients:

- 1 and ½ pounds beets, peeled and quartered
- A drizzle of olive oil
- 2 teaspoons orange zest, grated
- 2 tablespoons cider vinegar
- ½ cup orange juice
- 2 tablespoons brown sugar
- 2 scallions, chopped
- 2 teaspoons mustard
- 2 cups arugula

Directions:

1. Rub beets with the oil and orange juice, place them in your air fryer and cook at 350 degrees F for 10 minutes.
2. Transfer beet quarters to a bowl, add scallions, arugula and orange zest and toss.
3. In a separate bowl, mix sugar with mustard and vinegar, whisk well, add to salad, toss and serve.

Enjoy!

Nutrition: calories 121, fat 2, fiber 3, carbs 11, protein 4

Beet , Tomato and Goat Cheese Mix

Preparation time: 30 minutes **Cooking time:** 14 minutes
Servings: 8

Ingredients:

- 8 small beets, trimmed, peeled and halved
- 1 red onion, sliced
- 4 ounces goat cheese, crumbled
- 1 tablespoon balsamic vinegar
- Salt and black pepper to the taste
- 2 tablespoons sugar
- 1 pint mixed cherry tomatoes, halved
- 2 ounces pecans
- 2 tablespoons olive oil

Directions:

1. Put beets in your air fryer, season them with salt and pepper, cook at 350 degrees F for 14 minutes and transfer to a salad bowl.
2. Add onion, cherry tomatoes and pecans and toss.
3. In another bowl, mix vinegar with sugar and oil, whisk well until sugar dissolves and add to salad.
4. Also add goat cheese, toss and serve.

Enjoy!

Nutrition: calories 124, fat 7, fiber 5, carbs 12, protein 6

Broccoli Salad

Preparation time: 10 minutes **Cooking time:** 8 minutes

Servings: 4

Ingredients:

- 1 broccoli head, florets separated
- 1 tablespoon peanut oil
- 6 garlic cloves, minced
- 1 tablespoon Chinese rice wine vinegar
- Salt and black pepper to the taste

Directions:

1. In a bowl, mix broccoli with salt, pepper and half of the oil, toss, transfer to your air fryer and cook at 350 degrees F for 8 minutes, shaking the fryer halfway.
2. Transfer broccoli to a salad bowl, add the rest of the peanut oil, garlic and rice vinegar, toss really well and serve.

Enjoy!

Nutrition: calories 121, fat 3, fiber 4, carbs 4, protein 4

Brussels Sprouts and Tomatoes Mix

Preparation time: 5 minutes **Cooking time:** 10 minutes

Servings: 4

Ingredients:

- 1 pound Brussels sprouts, trimmed
- Salt and black pepper to the taste
- 6 cherry tomatoes, halved
- ¼ cup green onions, chopped
- 1 tablespoon olive oil

Directions:

1. Season Brussels sprouts with salt and pepper, put them in your air fryer and cook at 350 degrees F for 10 minutes.
2. Transfer them to a bowl, add salt, pepper, cherry tomatoes, green onions and olive oil, toss well and serve.

Enjoy!

Nutrition: calories 121, fat 4, fiber 4, carbs 11, protein 4

Air Fryer Meat Recipes

Flavored Rib Eye Steak

Preparation time: 10 minutes **Cooking time:** 20 minutes
Servings: 4

Ingredients:

- 2 pounds rib eye steak
- Salt and black pepper to the taste
- 1 tablespoons olive oil

For the rub:

- 3 tablespoons sweet paprika
- 2 tablespoons onion powder
- 2 tablespoons garlic powder
- 1 tablespoon brown sugar
- 2 tablespoons oregano, dried
- 1 tablespoon cumin, ground
- 1 tablespoon rosemary, dried

Directions:

1. In a bowl, mix paprika with onion and garlic powder, sugar, oregano, rosemary, salt, pepper and cumin, stir and rub steak with this mix.
2. Season steak with salt and pepper, rub again with the oil, put in your air fryer and cook at 400 degrees F for 20 minutes, flipping them halfway.
3. Transfer steak to a cutting board, slice and serve with a side salad.

Enjoy!

Nutrition: calories 320, fat 8, fiber 7, carbs 22, protein 21

Chinese Steak and Broccoli

Preparation time: 45 minutes **Cooking time:** 12 minutes
Servings: 4

Ingredients:

- ¾ pound round steak, cut into strips
- 1 pound broccoli florets
- 1/3 cup oyster sauce
- 2 teaspoons sesame oil
- 1 teaspoon soy sauce
- 1 teaspoon sugar
- 1/3 cup sherry
- 1 tablespoon olive oil
- 1 garlic clove, minced

Directions:

1. In a bowl, mix sesame oil with oyster sauce, soy sauce, sherry and sugar, stir well, add beef, toss and leave aside for 30 minutes.
2. Transfer beef to a pan that fits your air fryer, also add broccoli, garlic and oil, toss everything and cook at 380 degrees F for 12 minutes.
3. Divide among plates and serve.

Enjoy!

Nutrition: calories 330, fat 12, fiber 7, carbs 23, protein 23

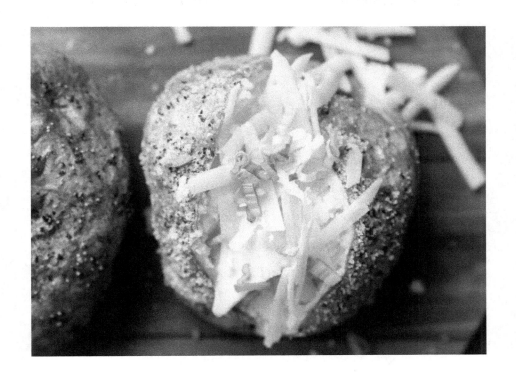

Provencal Pork

Preparation time: 10 minutes **Cooking time:** 15 minutes
Servings: 2

Ingredients:

- 1 red onion, sliced
- 1 yellow bell pepper, cut into strips
- 1 green bell pepper, cut into strips
- Salt and black pepper to the taste
- 2 teaspoons Provencal herbs
- ½ tablespoon mustard
- 1 tablespoon olive oil
- 7 ounces pork tenderloin

Directions:

1. In a baking dish that fits your air fryer, mix yellow bell pepper with green bell pepper, onion, salt, pepper, Provencal herbs and half of the oil and toss well.
2. Season pork with salt, pepper, mustard and the rest of the oil, toss well and add to veggies.
3. Introduce everything in your air fryer, cook at 370 degrees F for 15 minutes, divide among plates and serve.

Enjoy!

Nutrition: calories 300, fat 8, fiber 7, carbs 21, protein 23

Beef S trips with Snow Peas and Mushrooms

Preparation time: 10 minutes **Cooking time:** 22 minutes
Servings: 2

Ingredients:

- 2 beef steaks, cut into strips
- Salt and black pepper to the taste
- 7 ounces snow peas
- 8 ounces white mushrooms, halved
- 1 yellow onion, cut into rings
- 2 tablespoons soy sauce
- 1 teaspoon olive oil

Directions:

1. In a bowl, mix olive oil with soy sauce, whisk, add beef strips and toss.
2. In another bowl, mix snow peas, onion and mushrooms with salt, pepper and the oil, toss well, put in a pan that fits your air fryer and cook at 350 degrees F for 16 minutes.
3. Add beef strips to the pan as well and cook at 400 degrees F for 6 minutes more.
4. Divide everything on plates and serve.

Enjoy!

Nutrition: calories 235, fat 8, fiber 2, carbs 22, protein 24

Garlic Lamb Chops

Preparation time: 10 minutes **Cooking time:** 10 minutes
Servings: 4

Ingredients:

- 3 tablespoons olive oil
- 8 lamb chops
- Salt and black pepper to the taste
- 4 garlic cloves, minced
- 1 tablespoon oregano, chopped
- 1 tablespoon coriander, chopped

Directions:

1. In a bowl, mix oregano with salt, pepper, oil, garlic and lamb chops and toss to coat.
2. Transfer lamb chops to your air fryer and cook at 400 degrees F for 10 minutes.
3. Divide lamb chops on plates and serve with a side salad.

Enjoy!

Nutrition: calories 231, fat 7, fiber 5, carbs 14, protein 23

Crispy Lamb

Preparation time: 10 minutes **Cooking time:** 30 minutes

Servings: 4

Ingredients:

- 1 tablespoon bread crumbs
- 2 tablespoons macadamia nuts, toasted and crushed
- 1 tablespoon olive oil
- 1 garlic clove, minced
- 28 ounces rack of lamb
- Salt and black pepper to the taste
- 1 egg,
- 1 tablespoon rosemary, chopped

Directions:

1. In a bowl, mix oil with garlic and stir well.

2. Season lamb with salt, pepper and brush with the oil.

3. In another bowl, mix nuts with breadcrumbs and rosemary.

4. Put the egg in a separate bowl and whisk well.

5. Dip lamb in egg, then in macadamia mix, place them in your air fryer's basket, cook at 360 degrees F and cook for 25 minutes, increase heat to 400 degrees F and cook for 5 minutes more.

6. Divide among plates and serve right away.

Enjoy!

Nutrition: calories 230, fat 2, fiber 2, carbs 10, protein 12

Indian Pork

Preparation time: 35 minutes **Cooking time:** 10 minutes
Servings: 4

Ingredients:
- 1 teaspoon ginger powder
- 2 teaspoons chili paste
- 2 garlic cloves, minced
- 14 ounces pork chops, cubed
- 1 shallot, chopped
- 1 teaspoon coriander, ground
- 7 ounces coconut milk
- 2 tablespoons olive oil
- 3 ounces peanuts, ground
- 3 tablespoons soy sauce
- Salt and black pepper to the taste

Directions:

1. In a bowl, mix ginger with 1 teaspoon chili paste, half of the garlic, half of the soy sauce and half of the oil, whisk, add meat, toss and leave aside for 10 minutes.
2. Transfer meat to your air fryer's basket and cook at 400 degrees F for 12 minutes, turning halfway.
3. Meanwhile, heat up a pan with the rest of the oil over medium high heat, add shallot, the rest of the garlic, coriander, coconut milk, the rest of the peanuts, the rest of the chili paste and the rest of the soy sauce, stir and cook for 5 minutes.
4. Divide pork on plates, spread coconut mix on top and serve.

Enjoy!

Nutrition: calories 423, fat 11, fiber 4, carbs 42, protein 18

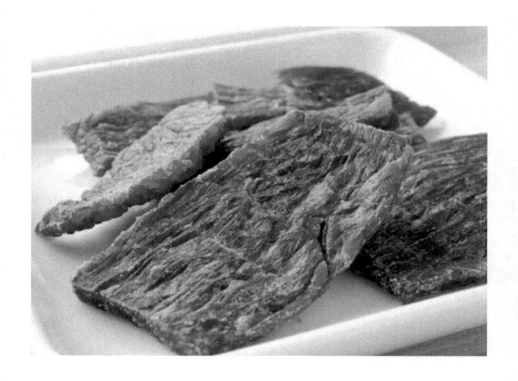

Lamb and Creamy Brussels Sprouts

Preparation time: 10 minutes **Cooking time:** 1 hour and 10 minutes **Servings:** 4

Ingredients:

- 2 pounds leg of lamb, scored
- 2 tablespoons olive oil
- 1 tablespoon rosemary, chopped
- 1 tablespoon lemon thyme, chopped
- 1 garlic clove, minced
- 1 and ½ pounds Brussels sprouts, trimmed
- 1 tablespoon butter, melted
- ½ cup sour cream
- Salt and black pepper to the taste

Directions:

1. Season leg of lamb with salt, pepper, thyme and rosemary, brush with oil, place in your air fryer's basket, cook at 300 degrees F for 1 hour, transfer to a plate and keep warm.
2. In a pan that fits your air fryer, mix Brussels sprouts with salt, pepper, garlic, butter and sour cream, toss, put in your air fryer and cook at 400 degrees F for 10 minutes.
3. Divide lamb on plates, add Brussels sprouts on the side and serve.

Enjoy!

Nutrition: calories 440, fat 23, fiber 0, carbs 2, protein 49

Beef Fillets with Garlic Mayo

Preparation time: 10 minutes **Cooking time:** 40 minutes
Servings: 8

Ingredients:

- 1 cup mayonnaise
- 1/3 cup sour cream
- 2 garlic cloves, minced
- 3 pounds beef fillet
- 2 tablespoons chives, chopped
- 2 tablespoons mustard
- 2 tablespoons mustard
- ¼ cup tarragon, chopped
- Salt and black pepper to the taste

Directions:

1. Season beef with salt and pepper to the taste, place in your air fryer, cook at 370 degrees F for 20 minutes, transfer to a plate and leave aside for a few minutes.
2. In a bowl, mix garlic with sour cream, chives, mayo, some salt and pepper, whisk and leave aside.

3. In another bowl, mix mustard with Dijon mustard and tarragon, whisk, add beef, toss, return to your air fryer and cook at 350 degrees F for 20 minutes more.

4. Divide beef on plates, spread garlic mayo on top and serve.

Enjoy!

Nutrition: calories 400, fat 12, fiber 2, carbs 27, protein 19

Mustard Marina ted Beef

Preparation time: 10 minutes **Cooking time:** 45 minutes

Servings: 6

Ingredients:

- 6 bacon strips
- 2 tablespoons butter
- 3 garlic cloves, minced
- Salt and black pepper to the taste
- 1 tablespoon horseradish
- 1 tablespoon mustard
- 3 pounds beef roast
- 1 and ¾ cup beef stock
- ¾ cup red wine

Directions:

1. In a bowl, mix butter with mustard, garlic, salt, pepper and horseradish, whisk and rub beef with this mix.
2. Arrange bacon strips on a cutting board, place beef on top, fold bacon around beef, transfer to your air fryer's basket, cook at 400 degrees F for 15 minutes and transfer to a pan that fits your fryer.

3. Add stock and wine to beef, introduce pan in your air fryer and cook at 360 degrees F for 30 minutes more.
4. Carve beef, divide among plates and serve with a side salad.

Enjoy!

Nutrition: calories 500, fat 9, fiber 4, carbs 29, protein 36

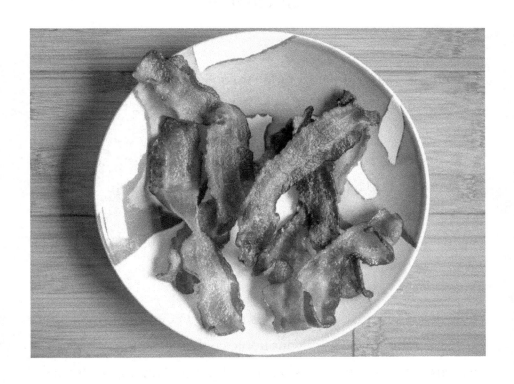

Conclusion

Air frying is one of the most popular cooking methods these days and air fryers have become one of the most amazing tools in the kitchen.

Air fryers help you cook healthy and delicious meals in no time! You don't need to be an expert in the kitchen in order to cook special dishes for you and your loved ones!

You just have to own an air fryer and this great air fryer cookbook!

You will soon make the best dishes ever and you will impress everyone around you with your home cooked meals!

Just trust us! Get your hands on an air fryer and on this useful air fryer recipes collection and start your new cooking experience! Have fun!

CPSIA information can be obtained
at www.ICGtesting.com
Printed in the USA
LVHW021022080621
689681LV00015B/1457